Contents

©1993, 1997, American Heart Association   ISBN 0-87493-614-4

Written material alone does not constitute a CPR course. To gain the skills of CPR, it is useful to practice on manikins with properly trained instructors as guides. Instructional videos may further enhance your skills.

Introduction

One of the most startling ideas of modern medicine is that "sudden death" can be reversed. Perhaps more astonishing is the realization that this miracle of science may be brought about *by any of us, anywhere,* using only our hands, our lungs, and our brains. Cardiopulmonary resuscitation (CPR) performed properly and promptly can help victims survive to receive treatment with advanced medical techniques.

This student manual is based on the latest information available. It will help you learn how your heart and circulatory system work and how that knowledge may help you avoid a heart attack through a sensible, prudent lifestyle. You will learn how to recognize warning signs of heart attack and stroke and what to do if they occur. You will also learn how to treat respiratory distress and choking (foreign-body airway obstruction).

Why Should I Learn CPR?

If you are reading this book, you have probably already made the commitment to learn how to perform CPR. Perhaps someone you love is suffering from heart disease. Maybe the nature of your job requires that you be prepared to handle medical emergencies. Or you may believe, as many people do, that knowing the skills of CPR simply makes you a more useful member of your community.

Whatever your reasons, it is important to remember that *CPR can help save lives.* Your hard work and study can make a difference. In 1990 cardiovascular disease accounted for more than 900 000 deaths, including nearly 500 000 due to heart attack. About two thirds of deaths from heart attack occur before the victim reaches the hospital. Many of these deaths can be prevented if the victims get prompt help — if someone trained in CPR provides proper life-saving measures until trained professionals take over.

After cardiac arrest, promptly initiated CPR may return victims to productive life. Without CPR, permanent brain death due to a lack of oxygen will occur. *Speed* in getting specialized medical care for victims and in starting CPR is the key to saving lives.

Chain of Survival

CPR *alone* is not enough to save lives in most cardiac arrests. It is, however, a vital link in the chain of survival that must be initiated to support the victim until other, more advanced support is available. The chain of survival includes the following sequence: early activation of the emergency medical services (EMS) system, early CPR, early defibrillation, and early advanced care.

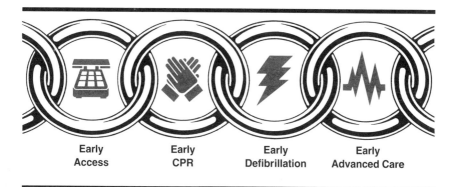

| Early Access | Early CPR | Early Defibrillation | Early Advanced Care |

You are vital to the success of the chain of survival because the first two links — early activation ("Call 911") and early CPR — will be in your hands. Early defibrillation and early advanced care will be provided by skilled emergency personnel who will respond *after your phone call.* Effective emergency cardiac care depends on strong interaction between all four parts of this chain. If any link is weak or missing, the chance of survival is lessened.

Early Access ("Call 911")

First, you, the bystander, must recognize the emergency. Recognizing the early warning signs of a heart attack and stroke, trying to prevent complications, and reassuring the victim are the initial steps in definitive care.

As soon as an emergency is recognized, the bystander (or victim, if able) must make a telephone call to activate the EMS system. This is sometimes referred to as "Phone First!" It is modified slightly for children to "Phone Fast!" (See the back cover for a place to record the telephone number of your local community rescue unit.) When you telephone for help, tell the operator:

1. *Where* the emergency is, with the address or names of cross streets, roads, or other landmarks if possible
2. *Telephone number* that you are calling from
3. *What happened* — heart attack, auto accident, fall, etc
4. *How many* persons need help
5. *Condition* of the victim(s)
6. *What* is being done for the victim(s)

You hang up last. Let the person you called hang up first.

In many areas of the country a specially trained dispatcher will instruct you on the next steps to help with the rescue.

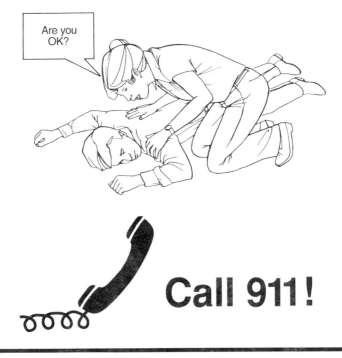

Early CPR

In this course you will learn how to do CPR:

- When and how to provide rescue breathing that will deliver air to the lungs of a victim suffering from respiratory arrest
- When and how to provide chest compressions that will circulate the blood of a victim suffering from cardiac arrest

Early Defibrillation

Early access to the EMS system will ensure that emergency personnel will arrive quickly, equipped with a defibrillator, a machine that delivers electric shocks to the heart. In the sudden cardiac arrest of an adult the most frequent initial abnormal heart rhythm is called *ventricular fibrillation.* This is an abnormal, chaotic heart rhythm that prevents the heart from pumping blood. The most effective treatment for this abnormal heart rhythm is defibrillation.

The earlier this shock is provided, the more likely the victim's life can be saved. In many communities throughout the United States many lives have been saved when early defibrillation programs have been started.

To learn more about early defibrillation, see Appendix 5: "Public Access Defibrillation and Automated External Defibrillators."

Early Advanced Care

Early advanced care includes basic life support measures plus more specialized care, which may be provided by doctors, nurses, paramedics, or other appropriately trained rescuers.

Normal Heart and Lung Anatomy and Function

    The heart is a muscle about the size of a clenched fist. It is located in the center of the chest behind the breastbone (sternum) and in front of the spine. The coronary arteries (not shown) are special arteries that supply blood to the heart muscle itself.

Location of the Heart

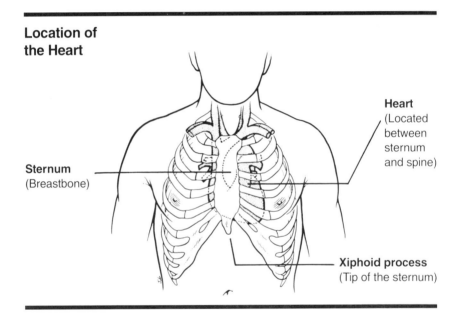

Heart
(Located between sternum and spine)

Sternum
(Breastbone)

Xiphoid process
(Tip of the sternum)

The Heart and Circulatory System

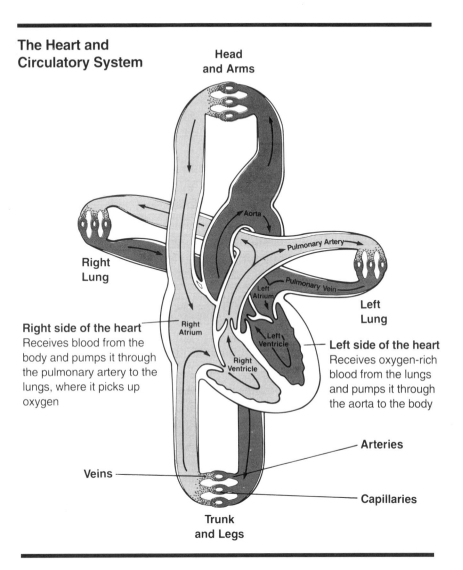

Head and Arms

Right Lung

Aorta

Pulmonary Artery

Pulmonary Vein

Left Atrium

Right Atrium

Left Ventricle

Right Ventricle

Left Lung

Right side of the heart
Receives blood from the body and pumps it through the pulmonary artery to the lungs, where it picks up oxygen

Left side of the heart
Receives oxygen-rich blood from the lungs and pumps it through the aorta to the body

Arteries

Veins

Capillaries

Trunk and Legs

The function of the heart is to pump blood to the lungs, where it picks up oxygen, and then to the rest of the body, where it delivers the oxygen. The adult heart pumps approximately 5 quarts (5 liters) of blood per minute. All cells of the body require oxygen to carry out their normal functions. When the heart stops pumping (cardiac arrest), oxygen is not circulated, and the oxygen stored in the brain and other vital organs is used quickly. The heartbeat is triggered by natural electrical impulses sent through the heart 60 to 100 times per minute in the healthy, resting adult. During exercise the heart of the average person can pump up to 25½ quarts (25 liters) each minute.

The lungs consist of many tiny air sacs (alveoli) surrounded by small blood vessels (capillaries). Nerve impulses from the brain to the chest muscles and the diaphragm cause a person to breathe. With each breath, air is carried through the **airway** (nose, mouth, throat, larynx, trachea, and bronchi) and into the air sacs of the lungs.

Parts of the Airway

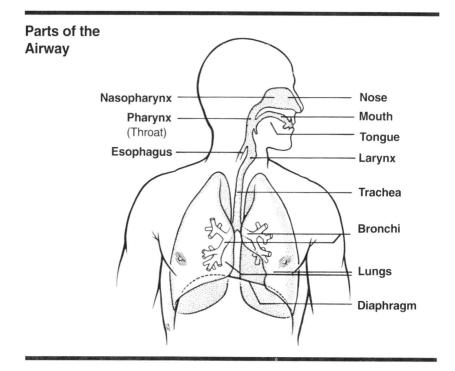

At sea level, approximately 21% of air is oxygen. When the air sacs fill with this air, oxygen enters the blood in the vessels surrounding the air sacs. The oxygenated blood returns to the heart, which pumps it throughout the body. As oxygen is taken from the blood by cells in the body, carbon dioxide is given off as a waste product. Carbon dioxide is carried by the blood to the air sacs and is exhaled out of the body. When air is inhaled, only one fourth of the oxygen is taken up by the blood; the rest is exhaled. This is why mouth-to-mouth breathing can provide the victim with enough oxygen.

When breathing stops (respiratory arrest), the heart continues to pump blood for several minutes, carrying existing stores of oxygen to the brain and the rest of the body. Early, prompt rescue efforts for the victim of respiratory arrest or choking (foreign-body airway obstruction) can often prevent the heart from stopping (cardiac arrest).

Coronary Artery Disease

Coronary artery disease affects the arteries that supply blood to the heart muscle. It is caused most often by **atherosclerosis,** which is the gradual buildup of fatty deposits on the inner lining of the artery walls. Atherosclerosis progressively narrows the artery and decreases the blood flow. This process may be compared to the gradual buildup of lime deposits in a pipe that finally plug the pipe completely. The disease may involve the arteries in many different areas of the body, including the heart (leading to a heart attack) and the brain (leading to a stroke). When the blood flow is severely reduced by atherosclerosis, a clot can form as blood trickles through the narrowed vessel, causing a sudden, complete stoppage of blood flow.

Atherosclerosis

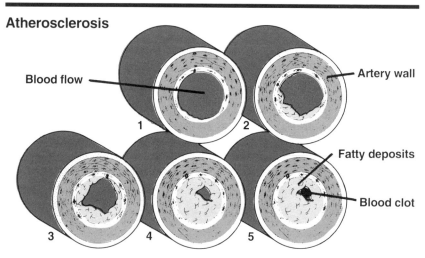

Blood flow — Artery wall

Fatty deposits

Blood clot

1 2 3 4 5

Progressive atherosclerotic buildup on artery walls. Atherosclerosis is commonly called *hardening of the arteries.* In atherosclerosis the inner lining (wall) of the artery becomes thickened and roughened by fatty deposits of cholesterol and other material. With the channels thus narrowed, blood supply is reduced. A blood clot can completely block the narrowed artery, resulting in death of the heart muscle cells supplied by that artery.

The process of atherosclerosis usually begins at an early age. Considerable disease may be present in some persons before age 20. The development of atherosclerosis can be hastened by certain risk factors: smoking, obesity, diabetes, inactivity, high blood pressure. Long before the function of the heart is affected, there is a period without symptoms. The narrowing progresses slowly. Modification of the risk factors noted above may halt or even reverse the process of atherosclerosis. Risk factors are discussed in greater detail on page 13.

Coronary artery disease may show up in three common ways — angina, heart attack, and sudden death.

- **Angina:** Some persons with coronary artery disease may experience temporary chest pressure or pain that is relieved by rest or nitroglycerin. This condition is known as *angina pectoris.* It occurs when narrowing of the coronary artery temporarily prevents an adequate supply of blood and oxygen to meet the demands of the working heart muscle. Once the demands of the heart muscle decrease, the pain disappears and there is usually no permanent damage to the heart muscle.

- **Heart attack:** A heart attack usually occurs when a blood clot suddenly and completely blocks a diseased coronary artery, resulting in the death of the heart muscle cells supplied by that artery. *Acute myocardial infarction* means "death of the heart muscle" due to inadequate blood supply and is another term for heart attack. *Coronary* and *coronary thrombosis* are commonly used terms for a heart attack. New drugs that dissolve blood clots can limit a heart attack in progress, but they must be administered as quickly as possible after the onset of symptoms. Maximum benefit occurs if the drugs can be given in the first hour. There may be some benefit from treatment as long as 6 to 12 hours after onset of heart attack symptoms.

- **Sudden cardiac death:** Sudden cardiac death due to cardiac arrest may, in many persons, be the first sign of coronary artery disease. In a cardiac arrest the heart stops pumping. When the heart stops, the victim will also stop breathing. Sudden death may occur as a complication of a heart attack, most commonly within 1 to 2 hours after the beginning of heart attack symptoms. More often it occurs independent of a heart attack. But in this kind of death, underlying atherosclerotic heart disease is usually present. Other causes of sudden death are listed below.

Common Causes of Sudden Death

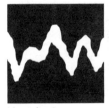

Ventricular
fibrillation

Accidental
electric shock

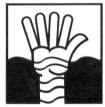

Drowning

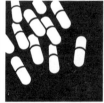

Drug
overdose

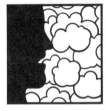

Suffocation

Severe allergic
reactions

Trauma

Stroke

At present fewer than 20% of people who experience sudden cardiac death are resuscitated. The key to improved outcome for these victims is you, the bystander. If you recognize the emergency and initiate the chain of survival (by calling EMS and then starting CPR), the chance of survival for such people can be improved.

Risk Factors for Heart Attack

Several factors increase a person's chances of having a heart attack. Some risk factors can be changed or controlled; others cannot. Risk factors for heart attack are listed below.

The danger of heart attack increases with the number of risk factors — the more risk factors present, the greater the risk. Reducing risk factors, however, can slow down arterial disease and even reverse it.

Men have an increased risk of heart attack. But it is important for women to control changeable risk factors as well. A woman's chance of dying after a heart attack is greater than a man's, and heart disease is the leading cause of death in women.

Major Risk Factors That Cannot Be Changed

- Heredity
- Male gender
- Increasing age

Major Risk Factors That Can Be Changed

- Cigarette smoke
- High blood pressure
- Blood cholesterol levels
- Physical inactivity

Other Contributing Factors

- Diabetes*
- Obesity
- Stress

* Elevated blood sugar levels associated with diabetes can be controlled, but the increased risk of heart disease cannot be eliminated.

Prudent Heart Living: *You* Are in Control

Prudent heart living is a lifestyle that may minimize the risk of future heart disease. Too many adult Americans are overweight, lead sedentary lives, and smoke heavily. Many have high levels of cholesterol and other fatty substances in their blood, and high blood pressure is common. Millions of Americans develop unhealthy living habits during childhood. These endanger the heart throughout life. Some children begin early in life to overeat and to develop a taste for foods high in cholesterol and calories. Some children do not get enough exercise (for example, they may watch too much television). Smoking frequently begins in the early teens, and children are more likely to smoke if their parents do.

Reducing risk factors may reduce the risk of having a heart attack or stroke. At the very least, reducing the risks can result in good general health and physical fitness and can benefit every member of the family. Children stand to benefit most by learning the habits of prudent heart living early in life.

The following pages describe in detail five specific ways that prudent heart living can be established and maintained.

1. Cigarette Smoking: DON'T

Exposure to cigarette smoke is the most important single cause of preventable death in the United States. Cigarette smokers have a greater risk of dying from a variety of diseases than do nonsmokers, and they have more than twice the risk of heart attack and two to four times the risk of sudden cardiac death.

If you have been a heavy smoker, will it help to stop now? Yes. People who quit smoking have a rapidly reduced risk of heart disease, and after a period of years their death rate is nearly as low as that of people who never smoked.

The earlier a person begins to smoke or use tobacco in any form, the greater the risk to future health. There is considerable peer pressure on teenagers to use tobacco, and whether they resist may depend largely on the example set by their parents.

Inhalation of environmental tobacco smoke, that is, *passive smoking,* has also been associated with an increased risk of smoking-related disease. Public buildings, hospitals, and many restaurants and businesses have implemented firm nonsmoking policies. These efforts encourage their patrons and employees to recognize risks for both active and passive smokers. Ongoing efforts in this public health area should lead to a decrease in the number of deaths and disability from cigarette smoking.

2. Control High Blood Pressure

Uncontrolled high blood pressure (hypertension) is associated with a greater risk of heart attack. When hypertension is not treated, it becomes a major health problem, and the result may be damage to blood vessels in the heart, kidneys, and other organs. High blood pressure increases the risk of stroke, heart attack, and kidney failure. When high blood pressure is combined with other risk factors, such as obesity, exposure to cigarette smoke, high blood cholesterol levels, physical inactivity, or diabetes, the risk of heart attack or stroke is greatly increased.

The underlying cause of high blood pressure in most patients is still unknown. However, high blood pressure is usually controllable. Treatment includes diet changes and increased exercise. Drugs to lower the blood pressure may be used if diet and exercise are in-effective. This is one of the most important reasons for having regular medical checkups: people who know they have high blood pressure can guard against its most harmful effects.

3. Reduce Saturated Fat and Cholesterol in the Diet

Cholesterol is a substance manufactured by our bodies. It is also present in the foods we eat. It is found in all animal products and is especially high in egg yolks and organ meats (liver, kidneys, brains). When excess cholesterol is deposited on the inner walls of arteries, it leads to a narrowing of the blood vessels known as atherosclerosis.

Saturated fats, such as those in red meats, butter, cheeses, cream, and whole milk, also seem to help raise the blood's choles-terol level. On the other hand, partially substituting polyunsaturated fats (such as liquid vegetable oils, with the exception of coconut, palm, and palm kernel oil, which are saturated fats) lowers choles-terol levels in most people. The goal is to keep the saturated fat content of the diet low. You cannot eliminate saturated fat entirely. It is present in many of the foods you eat. However, you can reduce the amount of saturated fat in your diet if you follow these recommendations:

- Have fish and poultry instead of red meat at most of your meals. Cook poultry without the skin. When you serve red meat (beef, pork, lamb), use lean cuts, trim off excess fat, and serve small portions.
- Cook with limited amounts of liquid vegetable oils and polyunsaturated margarines, such as canola, corn, soybean, and safflower products.
- Use skim-milk products.
- Eat no more than three egg yolks per week. Use "egg substitutes" (no-cholesterol alternatives) if possible.
- Use low-fat cooking methods, such as baking, broiling, and roasting. Avoid fried foods.

Dietary change should never be drastic. You can harm yourself by cutting out essential foods. Fad diets can lead to other health problems. However, with moderate changes in your diet, regular exercise, and careful attention to your intake of cholesterol and saturated fats, you can usually keep blood cholesterol down to normal levels.

4. Exercise Regularly

Evidence suggests that men who lead sedentary lives may have a higher risk of heart attack than those who get regular, vigorous exercise. Exercise tones the muscles, stimulates the circulation, helps prevent excess weight, and promotes a general feeling of well-being. The survival rate of heart attack victims is higher in those who have exercised regularly than in those who have not.

This does not mean that you should shovel snow in winter or play a hard game of tennis if you are not used to such exertion. Before starting an exercise program or heavy physical labor, consult your physician. He or she may suggest an exercise test to evaluate your physical condition. When participating in an exercise program, you should always increase your physical activity gradually.

You cannot go wrong, at least, by walking briskly when it is not absolutely necessary to ride. And you may want to take up a sport you will enjoy if your doctor says you are fit for it.

5. Weight Control: Count Your Calories

Most people reach their normal adult weight between the ages of 21 and 25. With each year after that, fewer calories are needed to maintain this weight. But people in their 30s and 40s often eat as much as they did in their early 20s, and if they become less active, the excess calories are stored as fat.

Life expectancy may be shorter for people who are overweight. Middle-aged men who are much overweight, for example, have about three times the risk of a fatal heart attack as middle-aged men of normal weight. Obesity also increases the risk of high blood pressure, high cholesterol, and diabetes.

There is no quick, easy way to reduce. It is best to avoid extreme reducing diets because they usually leave out foods essential to good health. Even when these diets lower weight, they do not help you develop eating habits that will keep weight normal. Controlling the fat in your diet may allow you to maintain an appropriate body weight. If you need to reduce, ask your doctor for advice.

Heart attack (or coronary heart disease) remains the No. 1 killer in the United States. Although we have a great deal more to do to save these lives, there has been a significant decline (49%) in age-adjusted death rates from coronary heart disease in the last 20 years. Several things have made this possible. One is drugs that provide better medical control of heart disease. Another is decreased risk from adoption of a healthful lifestyle (prudent heart living). Controlling risk factors *can* usually reduce cardiovascular mortality. Successful intervention at a young age is likely to have the greatest impact.

The American Heart Association publishes additional materials that can help you start prudent heart living. For more information, contact your local AHA.

How to Recognize a Heart Attack

Delay spells danger. When someone suffers a heart attack, minutes — especially the first few minutes — count. Know the signals!

Chest discomfort is the most common sign of a heart attack. It usually has the following characteristics:

What?　　Uncomfortable pressure, fullness, squeezing, or pain.

Where?　　In the center of the chest behind the breastbone. It may spread to, or occasionally originate in, either shoulder, the neck, the lower jaw, or either arm.

How long? The discomfort of a heart attack usually lasts longer than a few minutes. It may come and go.

Other signs of a heart attack may include any, all, or none of the following:

- Chest discomfort with lightheadedness
- Fainting
- Sweating
- Nausea
- Shortness of breath

Not all these warning signs occur in every heart attack. If some start to occur, however, don't wait. Get help immediately. Delay can be deadly!

Sharp, stabbing, short twinges of pain are usually *not* signals of a heart attack.

Many patients will deny that they may be having a heart attack. Expect these common reactions: "It's indigestion or something I ate" — "It can't happen to me" — "I'm too healthy" — "I don't want to bother the doctor" — "I'm under no strain" — "I don't want to frighten my wife/husband" — "I'll take a home remedy" — "I'll feel ridiculous if it isn't a heart attack." When the person starts looking for reasons why the illness cannot be a heart attack, this is a signal for positive action.

Because the victim may not act in his or her best interest, it is essential that the nearest person activate the EMS system and be prepared to perform CPR if necessary. If you are with someone who is having the signals of a heart attack and if they last longer than a few minutes, act at once.

The first step after activating the EMS system should be to have the victim rest quietly and calmly. Because both angina pectoris and heart attack are caused by too little oxygen to the heart muscle, the victim's activity and fear must be kept to a minimum. The victim should be allowed to assume the position that gives him or her the most comfort and allows the easiest breathing.

Stroke: Warning Signs and Risk Factors

Warning Signs of Stroke

Stroke is a common and serious brain illness of sudden onset. It results from the blockage or rupture of a blood vessel. Most often strokes are caused by a blood clot in an artery. *Stroke is a leading cause of death and disability among Americans.* Strokes may precipitate conditions that require rescue breathing, chest compressions, or both. Though most common in older people, *strokes happen in persons of all ages.* You should know the early warning signs of stroke so that emergency care can be started promptly. Warning signs or symptoms of stroke may include the following:

- Sudden weakness or numbness of the face, arm, or leg on one side of the body
- Loss of speech, slurred or incoherent speech
- Unexplained dizziness, unsteadiness, or sudden falls
- Dimness or loss of vision, particularly in one eye
- Loss of consciousness

An unusually severe or sudden intense headache ("the worst headache of my life") can be an important warning sign of a brain hemorrhage.

These warning signs may be temporary (a transient ischemic attack or TIA), lasting less than 24 hours or sometimes just a few minutes. *When one occurs, a physician should be sought immediately since prompt medical or surgical treatment can prevent a stroke.* If symptoms are severe, the EMS system should be activated. Although similar signs may result from alcohol or drug intoxication, insulin reactions, or other diseases, they may also be signs of stroke, even when temporary. Successful treatment of the victim is linked to early recognition, activation of the EMS system, and/or rapid transport to the hospital. The fundamentals of basic life support are important in the care of the patient with stroke, particularly when consciousness is impaired. Airway obstruction can occur.

If it does, immediately open the airway and perform rescue breathing.

Risk Factors for Stroke

Risk Factors That Cannot Be Controlled

Age: The incidence of stroke more than doubles every 10 years for people older than 55 years.

Gender: Men have a greater risk of stroke than women. Women who take oral contraceptives, especially if they also smoke, have a greater risk than other women.

Race: Black Americans have a greater risk of stroke than white Americans.

Diabetes mellitus

Prior stroke

Heredity

Risk Factors That Can Be Controlled

High blood pressure: High blood pressure (hypertension) is the most important risk factor for stroke because it affects one in every three Americans, yet it is usually readily controlled. The higher the blood pressure, the greater the risk. Much of the decline in the incidence of stroke is secondary to the improved management of high blood pressure.

Heart disease: A diseased heart can be both a defective (weak) pump and a source of blood clots. Some risk factors for coronary heart disease (elevated cholesterol level, cigarette smoking) are direct risk factors for stroke.

Cigarette smoking

High red blood cell count: An increase in the red blood cell count is a risk factor for stroke. The reason is that increased red blood cells thicken the blood and make clots more likely.

Transient ischemic attacks (TIAs): TIAs are strokelike symptoms that disappear in less than 24 hours. TIAs are extremely important; they are strong predictors of stroke. They are usually treated with drugs that help keep clots from forming.

Foreign-Body Airway Obstruction (Choking)

About 3800 deaths are reported to be caused by foreign-body airway obstruction (choking) every year. You will learn how to give first aid to victims of choking.

Causes

Choking usually occurs during eating. In adults, meat is the most common cause of obstruction, although a variety of foods and foreign bodies have been the cause of obstruction in children and some adults.

Risk Factors

- Large, poorly chewed pieces of food
- Elevated blood alcohol levels
- Dentures
- Playing, crying, laughing, or talking while food or foreign bodies are in the mouth

Prevention

- Cut food into small pieces and chew slowly and thoroughly, especially if you wear dentures.
- Avoid excessive intake of alcohol.
- Avoid laughing and talking while chewing and swallowing.
- Prevent children from playing, walking, or running with food or foreign objects in their mouths.
- Keep foreign objects (for example, marbles, beads, and thumb-tacks) away from infants and small children.

Recognition of Foreign-Body Airway Obstruction

Because early recognition of airway obstruction is the key to successful treatment, it is important to distinguish this emergency from fainting, stroke, heart attack, drug overdose, or other conditions that cause sudden respiratory failure but are managed differently.

Airway obstruction may also be due to infections that cause airway swelling. Children with an infectious cause of airway obstruction need prompt medical attention in a hospital's emergency department, and time should not be wasted on a futile attempt to relieve this kind of obstruction.

Foreign bodies may cause either partial or complete airway obstruction. With partial airway obstruction, the victim may be capable of either "good air exchange" or "poor air exchange." With good air exchange, the victim remains conscious and can cough forcefully, although frequently there is wheezing between coughs. With complete airway obstruction the victim is unable to speak, breathe, or cough.

Unrelieved airway obstruction will require professional help. Be sure to call your EMS system if you cannot clear the obstruction.

CPR Techniques

Early CPR is an important link in the chain of survival for a victim of sudden cardiac or respiratory arrest. CPR involves a combination of mouth-to-mouth rescue breathing (or other artificial ventilation techniques) and chest compressions. It keeps some oxygenated blood flowing to the brain and other vital organs until appropriate medical treatment can restore normal heart action.

Cardiac arrest causes the victim to lose consciousness within seconds. **If there is early access to the EMS system (Phone First! Phone Fast!), early CPR, early defibrillation, and early advanced care,** the person has a chance to survive.

CPR techniques include three basic rescue skills, the ABCs of CPR: Airway, Breathing, and Circulation.

Airway

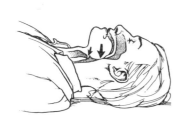

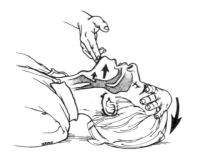

A key action for successful resuscitation is immediate opening of the airway by positioning the head properly. It is important to remember that the back of the tongue and the epiglottis are the most common causes of airway obstruction in the unconscious victim. Since the tongue, directly, and the epiglottis, indirectly, are attached to the lower jaw, tilting the head back and moving the lower jaw (chin) forward lifts the tongue and the epiglottis from the back of the throat and usually opens the airway.

Breathing

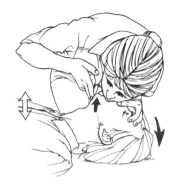

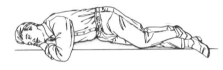

When breathing stops, the body has only the oxygen remaining in the lungs and bloodstream. Therefore, when breathing stops, cardiac arrest and death quickly follow. Mouth-to-mouth rescue breathing is the quickest way to get oxygen into the victim's lungs. There is more than enough oxygen in the air you breathe into the victim to supply the victim's needs. Rescue breathing should be performed until the victim can breathe on his or her own or until trained professionals take over.

• If the victim is unconscious and breathing and there is no evidence of trauma, you should place the victim on his or her side in the recovery position.

• If the victim's heart is beating, you should (1) maintain an open airway and (2) breathe for the victim.

• If the victim's heart is not beating, you should perform rescue breathing *plus* chest compressions.

Circulation

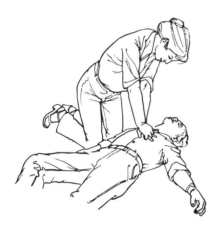

Chest compressions can maintain some blood flow to the lungs, brain, coronary arteries, and other major organs. When chest compressions are performed, rescue breathing should also be performed.

Recovery position:
If the victim resumes breathing and regains a pulse during or following resuscitation, you should place the victim in the recovery position.

Performance Guidelines and How to Use Them

Performance guidelines are presented in this section. They are designed to help you learn the basic emergency actions taught in your CPR course. They will give you the specific steps necessary to do the following:

- Perform CPR for a victim whose breathing and/or pulse have stopped (pp. 28–33)
- Clear a victim's airway if it is obstructed by foreign material (pp. 34–37)

This section contains pictures of each important step and a description of the step. Use this section:

- *Before* you take a CPR course to help you prepare for what is ahead
- *During* your CPR course, as you practice on a manikin, to guide your performance
- *After* you have finished the course to help refresh your memory

CPR, like any skill, must be practiced so that you can remember the important steps. That way, if an emergency arises, you may be able to help save a life. Renew your skills at least every 2 years by calling your local AHA and taking a refresher course. More frequent training is even better. It will take only a little time to review these emergency actions, and you will feel good knowing that you are still able to do CPR. A regular update also keeps you informed about advances in CPR technique.

Never rehearse or practice these skills on another person! They can be dangerous to a conscious, healthy person, but they are lifesaving for the cardiac arrest victim!

Performance Guidelines

	Action

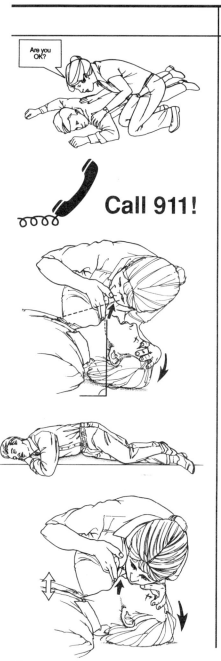	**Early Access**
	   Assessment: Determine unresponsiveness.
	
	Activate EMS System
	
	Early CPR
	Airway
	   Position the victim.
	
	   Open the airway (head tilt–chin lift).
	
	Breathing
	   Assessment: Determine breathlessness.
	
	   If the victim is breathing and there is no evidence of trauma, place the victim in the recovery position.
	
	   If the victim is not breathing, give 2 slow breaths ($1\frac{1}{2}$ to 2 seconds per breath).

Are you OK?

Call 911!

Helpful Hints

Tap or gently shake shoulder. Shout "Are you OK?"

Call 911 or your local emergency number. (Phone First!)

Turn on back if necessary, supporting head and neck.

Lift the chin up gently with one hand while pushing down on the forehead with the other to tilt the head back.

Look at the chest for movement.
Listen for the sounds of breathing.
Feel for breath on your cheek.

Place the victim on his or her side, using the victim's arm and leg for stabilization.

Pinch nostrils closed.

Make a tight seal around victim's mouth. Watch for victim's chest to rise.

Allow the lungs to deflate between breaths.

Performance Guidelines

	Action
	Circulation Assessment: Determine pulselessness.
	If the victim has a pulse, perform rescue breathing.
	If no pulse, begin first cycle of compressions and ventilations.
	15 compressions and 2 ventilations At the end of 4 cycles, check for return of pulse.

Helpful Hints

Place 2 or 3 fingers on the Adam's apple (voice box). Slide fingers into the groove between Adam's apple and muscle.
Feel for the carotid pulse.

Provide about 12 breaths per minute (1 breath every 5 seconds).

Find a position on the lower half of the sternum (breastbone).
Compress with weight transmitted downward.
Count to establish rhythm: "one and, two and, three and, four and…"
Depress the sternum 1½ to 2 inches, at a rate of 80 to 100 compressions per minute.

After every 15 compressions, deliver 2 slow rescue breaths.
If no pulse, resume CPR, starting with chest compressions.
If there is a pulse but no breathing, give 1 rescue breath every 5 seconds.

Performance Guidelines

Entrance of a Second Rescuer to Replace the First Rescuer

Second rescuer appears and

- Identifies himself or herself: "I know CPR. Can I help?"
- Asks if EMS has been activated and seeks help if necessary
- Checks pulse

If no pulse, second rescuer starts one-rescuer CPR and resumes the cycle of chest compressions and ventilations with as little interruption as possible.

First rescuer assesses the adequacy of second rescuer's efforts by

- Watching for chest to rise during rescue breaths
- Checking pulse during chest compressions

When the rescuer doing chest compressions and ventilations tires, the other rescuer should take over. The two rescuers should alternate roles until EMS arrives.

Performance Guidelines
Obstructed Airway: Conscious Adult

	Action
	Determine if victim is able to speak or cough.
	Abdominal thrust Perform the Heimlich maneuver until the foreign body is expelled or the victim becomes unconscious.
	Chest thrust *For victims who are in advanced pregnancy or who are obese*

Helpful Hints

Rescuer can ask "Are you choking?"
Victim may be using the "universal distress signal" of choking: clutching the neck between thumb and index finger.

Stand behind victim and wrap your arms around victim's waist. Press fist into abdomen with quick inward and upward thrusts.

Chest thrusts: Stand behind victim and place your arms under victim's armpits to encircle the chest. Press with quick backward thrusts.

Performance Guidelines

	Action
	Activate EMS.
	Check for foreign body.
	Attempt rescue breathing.
	If airway is obstructed, perform Heimlich maneuver.
	Repeat sequence until successful.

36

Helpful Hints

Call 911.

Sweep deeply into mouth with hooked finger to remove foreign body.

Open airway. Try to give 2 breaths. If needed, reposition the head and try again.

Kneel astride the victim's thighs. Place the heel of one hand on the victim's abdomen, in the midline slightly above the navel and well below the tip of the xiphoid. Place the second hand on top of the first. Press into the abdomen with quick upward thrusts.

Alternate these maneuvers in rapid sequence:
Finger sweep
Rescue breathing attempt
Abdominal thrusts

CPR and Airway Obstruction Management in Infants and Children

CPR and management of complete airway obstruction (first aid for choking) for children older than 8 years is the same as for adults. But treatment of airway obstruction in small children (1 to 8 years) and infants (less than 1 year) requires some changes from techniques used for adults. These differences in technique are necessary because of the small size and physical immaturity of infants and young children.

Because this course includes only an introduction to basic life support for infants and children, it is recommended that the following persons participate in a complete pediatric basic life support course:

- Parents of infants and young children, especially those at high risk for development of cardiorespiratory distress
- Day-care personnel
- Teachers
- Sports supervisors
- All healthcare personnel and professional rescuers

Causes of Sudden Death in Infants and Children

Cardiac arrest in infants and children is usually the result of lack of oxygen caused by respiratory difficulty or arrest. CPR in children may be required after a variety of events, such as injuries, airway obstruction caused by foreign objects (toys, foods, plastic covers, etc), near-drowning, smoke inhalation, sudden infant death syndrome, and infections.

Injuries and poisonings account for more than 8000 fatalities in children under age 15 every year. Nearly half of all injuries involve motor vehicle accidents, and about 20% involve burns, firearms, and poisoning.

Prevention

It is important to remember that time spent preventing conditions that cause cardiorespiratory deterioration in infants and children is much more productive than time spent mastering CPR techniques.

The majority of emergency situations requiring CPR are *preventable,* and special attention must be paid to making environments safe for children. Proper use of age-appropriate motor vehicle restraint devices (including child safety seats and seat belts) and bicycle helmets, installation of circumferential swimming pool barriers, proper safeguards for firearms in the home, and use of smoke detectors could prevent more than half of childhood injuries and half of all deaths caused by injuries. Children should be taught respect for matches and fires, and young children should not be left unsupervised. Items such as beads, small toys, thumbtacks, marbles, and peanuts must be kept away from infants and preschool children. Children should not have food or foreign objects in their mouths when they are walking, running, playing, or crying.

One-Rescuer CPR: Child (1 to 8 years)

CPR performed on young children is similar to CPR for adults and older children except for four differences:

1. If the rescuer has no help, give about 1 minute of CPR before activating the EMS system.
2. Use the heel of one hand in chest compressions rather than both hands.
3. Depress the sternum one third to one half the depth of the chest (about 1 to 1 1/2 inches).
4. Provide 100 compressions per minute, giving 1 rescue breath for every 5 chest compressions.

Remember that the numbers used in this section are broad guidelines.

Airway

1. *Assessment: Determine unresponsiveness.* Tap or gently shake shoulder and shout "Are you OK?"
2. *Call out "Help!"*
3. *Position the victim* on his or her back, taking care to support the head and neck in case of injury.
4. *Open the airway, using head tilt–chin lift.*

Breathing

5. *Assessment: Determine breathlessness.* With your ear over the child's mouth, look at the chest and *look, listen,* and *feel* for breath while keeping the airway open.

   If the victim is breathing and there is no evidence of trauma, *place the victim in the recovery position* (pp. 28–29).
6. If the victim is not breathing, *give 2 rescue breaths,* mouth to mouth (1 to 1 1/2 seconds per breath). The chest should rise with each breath, then fall.

Circulation

7. *Assessment: Determine pulselessness.* Using two or three fingers, feel for the carotid pulse with one hand while maintaining head tilt with the other.

8. *Begin chest compressions.* Find proper hand position as in adults. Compress the sternum approximately one third to one half the depth of the chest (this will be approximately 1 to 1½ inches, although these measurements are not precise). Use only the heel of one hand. 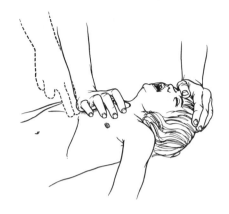 Compress the chest 100 times per minute, giving 1 rescue breath for every 5 compressions.

9. Do 20 cycles of compressions and rescue breaths.

10. *Activate the EMS system.* Call 911. (Phone Fast!)

11. Check pulse.

12. If no pulse, continue compressions and rescue breaths.

13. Check the pulse every few minutes.

14. If the pulse returns, check for spontaneous breathing. If there is no breathing, give 1 rescue breath every 3 seconds (20 rescue breaths per minute) and monitor the pulse. If the victim is breathing, place in the recovery position, maintain an open airway, and monitor breathing and pulse.

Entrance of Second Rescuer

1. Second rescuer arrives, identifies himself or herself, offers help, including activating the EMS if necessary, and checks pulse.

2. If no pulse, second rescuer takes over one-rescuer CPR.

3. First rescuer monitors second rescuer by (1) watching for the rise and fall of the chest during rescue breaths and (2) checking the pulse during chest compressions.

Obstructed Airway: Child (1 to 8 years)

Perform first aid for choking in children 1 to 8 years old just as you would for adults and older children, except do not perform blind finger sweeps. Instead, perform the tongue-jaw lift, look down into the airway, and use your finger to sweep the foreign body out only if you can actually see it.

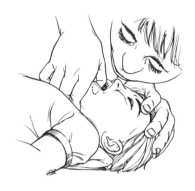

One-Rescuer CPR: Infant (less than 1 year)

CPR in infants must be performed with special consideration for size and vulnerabilities. For this reason there are several differences in CPR and first aid for choking in infants.

Airway

1. *Assessment: Determine unresponsiveness.* Tap or gently shake the shoulder.

2. *Call out "Help!"*

3. *Position the infant* on his or her back on a firm surface, supporting the head and neck if turning is necessary.

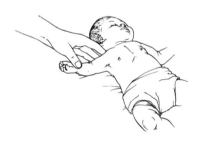

4. *Open the airway* using head tilt–chin lift. Take care not to tilt the head too far back.

Breathing

5. *Assessment: Determine breathlessness.* While maintaining an open airway, place your ear over the infant's mouth and *look* at the chest for movement, *listen* for breathing, and *feel* for breaths on your ear.

   If the victim is breathing and there is no evidence of trauma, *place the victim in the recovery position* (pp. 28–29).

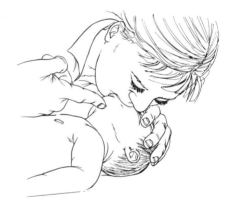

6. If the victim is not breathing, *give 2 gentle rescue breaths,* with your mouth covering the infant's mouth and nose, while maintaining an open airway. Observe the rise and fall of the chest. Each breath should be provided for 1 to 1^1/$_2$ seconds.

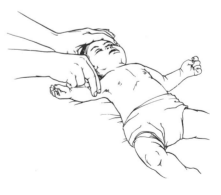

Circulation

7. *Assessment: Determine pulselessness.* Feel for the brachial pulse on the inside of the upper arm with two fingers of one hand while maintaining head tilt with the other hand.

8. *Begin chest compressions.* Imagine a line drawn between the nipples, and place your index finger below that line in the center of the chest. Place the middle and ring fingers next to the index finger. Use the middle and ring (third and fourth) fingers to compress the sternum at that point. Because of wide variations in the relative sizes of rescuers' hands and infants' chests, these instructions are only guidelines. After finding the position for compressions, make sure that you do not compress over the xiphoid process. Compress the sternum approximately one third to one half the depth of the chest (about $1/2$ to 1 inch) at least 100 times per minute. Give 1 rescue breath for every 5 compressions.

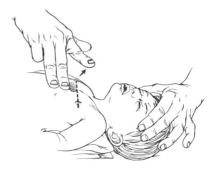

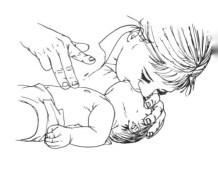

9. Do 20 cycles of compressions and rescue breaths.
10. *Activate the EMS system.* Call 911. (Phone Fast!)
11. Check the brachial pulse.
12. If no pulse, continue compressions and rescue breaths.
13. Feel for the pulse every few minutes.
14. If the pulse returns, check for spontaneous breathing. If there is no breathing, give 1 rescue breath every 3 seconds (20 rescue breaths per minute) and monitor the pulse. If there is breathing, place in the recovery position, maintain an open airway, and monitor breathing and pulse.

Obstructed Airway: Conscious Infant (less than 1 year)

Do not perform this procedure on a conscious infant unless complete airway obstruction is present (serious breathing difficulty, ineffective cough, *no* strong cry) and is due to a witnessed or strongly suspected obstruction by a foreign object. If obstruction is caused by swelling due to infection, the infant should be rushed to the nearest advanced life support facility, and maneuvers to clear the airway should *not* be performed. When respiratory distress is present, the infant should be allowed to find and maintain the position that he or she finds the most comfortable.

1. *Assessment: Determine airway obstruction.* Observe breathing difficulties, ineffective cough, weak (or absent) cry, dusky color.

2. *Place infant face down over one arm and deliver up to 5 back blows.* Supporting the head and neck with one hand, place the infant face down, head lower than trunk, over your forearm supported on your thigh. Deliver up to 5 back blows forcefully between the shoulder blades with the heel of one hand.

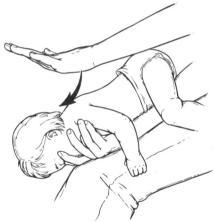

3. *Turn infant face up, supported on your arm, and deliver up to 5 chest thrusts.* Supporting the head, sandwich the infant between your hands/arms and turn on his or her back, head lower than trunk. Deliver up to 5 thrusts in the midsternal region, using the same landmarks as those for chest compressions.

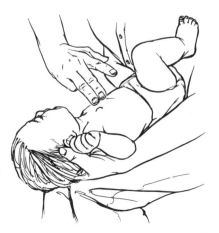

Deliver chest thrusts more slowly than when doing chest compressions.

4. Repeat steps 2 and 3 until either the foreign object is expelled or the infant becomes unconscious.

If the Infant Becomes Unconscious

5. *Call out "Help!"* If someone comes, that person should activate the EMS system. Position infant on back.

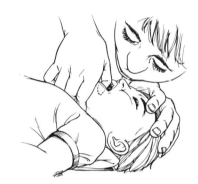

6. *Perform tongue-jaw lift.* Do not perform a blind finger sweep; remove foreign body only if you can see it.

7. *Try to give rescue breaths.* Open airway with head tilt–chin lift and try to give breaths.

8. *Try again to give rescue breaths.* Reposition the head and try to give rescue breaths.

9. *Deliver up to 5 back blows.*

10. *Deliver up to 5 chest thrusts.*

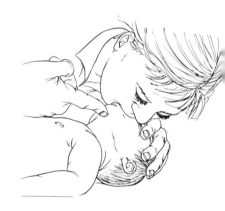

11. *Perform tongue-jaw lift* and remove foreign body if you see one.

12. *Try again to give rescue breaths,* while maintaining an open airway with head tilt–chin lift.

13. Repeat steps 8 through 12 until successful.

14. If you are alone and your efforts are unsuccessful, activate the EMS system after about 1 minute of efforts to clear the airway.

15. When obstruction is removed, check for breathing and pulse.

16. If there is breathing, place in the recovery position and monitor breathing and pulse while maintaining an open airway. If there is no breathing, give 20 rescue breaths per minute and monitor the pulse.

17. If no pulse, give 2 breaths and start cycles of compressions and breaths. If there is a pulse, open the airway and check for breathing.

Obstructed Airway: Unconscious Infant (less than 1 year)

1. *Assessment: Determine unresponsiveness* by tapping or gently shaking the shoulder.
2. *Call out "Help!"*
3. *Position the infant.* Turn on back, if necessary, on a firm, hard surface while supporting the head and neck.
4. *Open the airway.* Use head tilt–chin lift but take care not to tilt the head too far back.

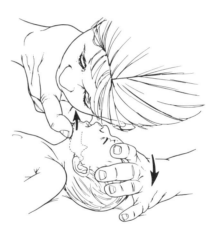

5. *Assessment: Determine breathlessness.* Maintaining an open airway, place your ear over the infant's mouth and *look* at the chest for breathing movement, *listen* for breathing sounds, and *feel* for breaths on your ear.
6. *Try to give rescue breaths.* Use a mouth-over-mouth-and-nose seal.
7. *Try again to give rescue breaths.* Reposition head and check mouth-over-mouth-and-nose seal.

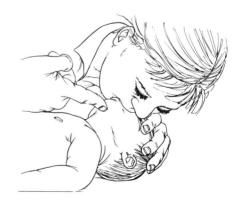

8. *Activate the EMS system.* If someone else is there, that person should activate the EMS system.

9. *Deliver up to 5 back blows.*

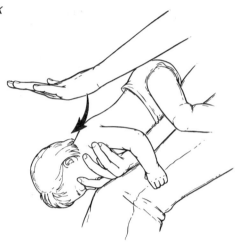

10. *Deliver up to 5 chest thrusts.*

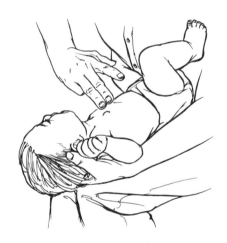

11. *Perform tongue-jaw lift* and remove foreign object if you see one.

12. *Try again to give rescue breaths. If unsuccessful, reposition head and try again.*

13. Repeat steps 9 through 12 until successful.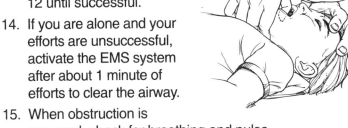

14. If you are alone and your efforts are unsuccessful, activate the EMS system after about 1 minute of efforts to clear the airway.

15. When obstruction is removed, check for breathing and pulse.

16. If there is breathing, place in the recovery position and monitor breathing and pulse while maintaining an open airway. If there is no breathing, give 20 rescue breaths per minute and monitor the pulse.

17. If no pulse, give 2 breaths and start cycles of compressions and breaths. If there is a pulse, open the airway and check for breathing.

Skill Performance Sheet
Adult One-Rescuer CPR

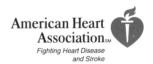

American Heart
Association℠
Fighting Heart Disease
and Stroke

Student Name _____ Date _____

Performance Guidelines	Performed
1. Establish unresponsiveness. Activate the EMS system.	
2. Open airway (head tilt–chin lift or jaw thrust). Check breathing (look, listen, feel).*	
3. Give 2 slow breaths (1½ to 2 seconds per breath), watch chest rise, allow for exhalation between breaths.	
4. Check carotid pulse. If breathing is absent but pulse is present, provide rescue breathing (1 breath every 5 seconds, about 12 breaths per minute).	
5. If no pulse, give cycles of 15 chest compressions (rate, 80 to 100 compressions per minute) followed by 2 slow breaths.	
6. After 4 cycles of 15:2 (about 1 minute), check pulse.* If no pulse, continue 15:2 cycle beginning with chest compressions.	

*If victim is breathing or resumes effective breathing, place in recovery position.

Comments _____

_____

_____

Instructor _____

Circle one: Complete   Needs more practice

Skill Performance Sheet
Adult Two-Rescuer CPR

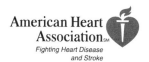

American Heart
Association_{SM}
*Fighting Heart Disease
and Stroke*

Student Name _____ Date _____

Performance Guidelines	Performed
1. Establish unresponsiveness. EMS system has been activated.	
RESCUER 1	
2. Open airway (head tilt–chin lift or jaw thrust). Check breathing (look, listen, feel).*	
3. Give 2 slow breaths (1½ to 2 seconds per breath), watch chest rise, allow for exhalation between breaths.	
4. Check carotid pulse.	
RESCUER 2	
5. If no pulse, give cycles of 5 chest compressions (rate, 80 to 100 compressions per minute) followed by 1 slow breath by Rescuer 1.	
6. After 1 minute of rescue support, check pulse.* If no pulse, continue 5:1 cycles.	

*If victim is breathing or resumes effective breathing, place in recovery position.

Comments _____

_____

_____

Instructor _____

Circle one: Complete   Needs more practice

Skill Performance Sheet
Adult Foreign-Body Airway Obstruction — Conscious

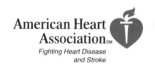

American Heart
Association℠

Fighting Heart Disease and Stroke

Student Name _____ Date _____

Performance Guidelines	Performed
1. Ask "Are you choking?"	
2. Give abdominal thrusts (chest thrusts for pregnant or obese victim).	
3. Repeat thrusts until effective or victim becomes unconscious.	
Adult Foreign-Body Airway Obstruction — Victim Becomes Unconscious	
4. Activate the EMS system.	
5. Perform a tongue-jaw lift followed by a finger sweep to remove the object.	
6. Open airway and try to ventilate; if still obstructed, reposition head and try to ventilate again.	
7. Give up to 5 abdominal thrusts.	
8. Repeat steps 5 through 7 until effective.*	

*If victim is breathing or resumes effective breathing, place in recovery position.

Comments _____

_____

_____

Instructor _____

Circle one:　　Complete　　Needs more practice

Skill Performance Sheet
Adult Foreign-Body Airway Obstruction — Unconscious

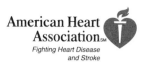
American Heart Association℠

Fighting Heart Disease and Stroke

Student Name _____ Date _____

Performance Guidelines	Performed
1. Establish unresponsiveness. Activate the EMS system.	
2. Open airway and try to ventilate; if still obstructed, reposition head and try to ventilate again.	
3. Give up to 5 abdominal thrusts.	
4. Perform a tongue-jaw lift followed by a finger sweep to remove the object.	
5. Repeat steps 2 through 4 until effective.*	

*If victim is breathing or resumes effective breathing, place in recovery position.

Comments _____ _____

_____

_____

Instructor _____

Circle one: Complete   Needs more practice

Skill Performance Sheet
Child One-Rescuer CPR

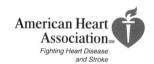

American Heart
Association℠

*Fighting Heart Disease
and Stroke*

Student Name _____ Date _____

Performance Guidelines	Performed
1. Establish unresponsiveness. If second rescuer is available, have him or her activate the EMS system.	
2. Open airway (head tilt–chin lift or jaw thrust). Check breathing (look, listen, feel).*	
3. Give 2 slow breaths (1 to 1½ seconds per breath), watch chest rise, allow for exhalation between breaths.	
4. Check carotid pulse. If breathing is absent but pulse is present, provide rescue breathing (1 breath every 3 seconds, about 20 breaths per minute).	
5. If no pulse, give 5 chest compressions (100 compressions per minute), open airway, and provide 1 slow breath. Repeat this cycle.	
6. After about 1 minute of rescue support, check pulse.* If rescuer is alone, activate the EMS system. If no pulse, continue 5:1 cycles.	

*If victim is breathing or resumes effective breathing, place in recovery position.

Comments _____

_____

_____

Instructor _____

Circle one: Complete   Needs more practice

Skill Performance Sheet
Child Foreign-Body Airway Obstruction — Conscious

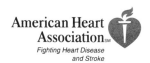

American Heart
Association℠
*Fighting Heart Disease
and Stroke*

Student Name _____ Date _____

Performance Guidelines	Performed
1. Ask "Are you choking?"	
2. Give abdominal thrusts.	
3. Repeat thrusts until effective or victim becomes unconscious.	
Child Foreign-Body Airway Obstruction — Victim Becomes Unconscious	
4. If second rescuer is available, have him or her activate the EMS system.	
5. Perform a tongue-jaw lift, and if you see the object, perform a finger sweep to remove it.	
6. Open airway and try to ventilate; if still obstructed, reposition head and try to ventilate again.	
7. Give up to 5 abdominal thrusts.	
8. Repeat steps 5 through 7 until effective.*	
9. If airway obstruction is not relieved after about 1 minute, activate the EMS system.	

*If victim is breathing or resumes effective breathing, place in recovery position.

Comments _____

_____

_____

Instructor _____

Circle one: Complete   Needs more practice

55

Skill Performance Sheet
Child Foreign-Body Airway Obstruction — Unconscious

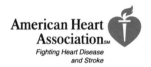

American Heart
Association℠
*Fighting Heart Disease
and Stroke*

Student Name _____ Date _____

Performance Guidelines	Performed
1. Establish unresponsiveness. If second rescuer is available, have him or her activate the EMS system.	
2. Open airway and try to ventilate; if still obstructed, reposition head and try to ventilate again.	
3. Give up to 5 abdominal thrusts.	
4. Perform a tongue-jaw lift, and if you see the object, perform a finger sweep to remove it.	
5. Repeat steps 2 through 4 until effective.*	
6. If airway obstruction is not relieved after about 1 minute, activate the EMS system.	

*If victim is breathing or resumes effective breathing, place in recovery position.

Comments _____

_____

_____

Instructor _____

Circle one: Complete   Needs more practice

Skill Performance Sheet
Infant One-Rescuer CPR

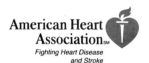

American Heart
Association_{SM}
Fighting Heart Disease
and Stroke

Student Name _____ Date _____

Performance Guidelines	Performed
1. Establish unresponsiveness. If second rescuer is available, have him or her activate the EMS system.	
2. Open airway (head tilt–chin lift or jaw thrust). Check breathing (look, listen, feel).*	
3. Give 2 slow breaths (1 to 1¹/₂ seconds per breath), watch chest rise, allow for exhalation between breaths.	
4. Check brachial pulse. If breathing is absent but pulse is present, provide rescue breathing (1 breath every 3 seconds, about 20 breaths per minute).	
5. If no pulse, give cycles of 5 chest compressions (rate, at least 100 compressions per minute) followed by 1 slow breath.	
6. After about 1 minute of rescue support, check pulse.* If rescuer is alone, activate the EMS system. If no pulse, continue 5:1 cycles.	

*If victim is breathing or resumes effective breathing, place in recovery position.

Comments _____

_____

_____

Instructor _____

Circle one: Complete   Needs more practice

Skill Performance Sheet
Infant Foreign-Body Airway Obstruction — Conscious

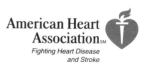

American Heart
Association℠
*Fighting Heart Disease
and Stroke*

Student Name _____ Date _____

Performance Guidelines	Performed
1. Confirm complete airway obstruction. Check for serious breathing difficulty, ineffective cough, *no* strong cry.	
2. Give up to 5 back blows and 5 chest thrusts.	
3. Repeat step 2 until effective or victim becomes unconscious.	
Infant Foreign-Body Airway Obstruction — Victim Becomes Unconscious	
4. If second rescuer is available, have him or her activate the EMS system.	
5. Perform a tongue-jaw lift, and if you see the object, perform a finger sweep to remove it.	
6. Open airway and try to ventilate; if still obstructed, reposition head and try to ventilate again.	
7. Give up to 5 back blows and 5 chest thrusts.	
8. Repeat steps 5 through 7 until effective.*	
9. If airway obstruction is not relieved after about 1 minute, activate the EMS system.	

*If victim is breathing or resumes effective breathing, place in recovery position.

Comments _____

_____

_____

Instructor _____

Circle one: Complete   Needs more practice

Skill Performance Sheet
Infant Foreign-Body Airway Obstruction — Unconscious

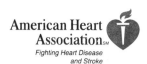

American Heart
Association℠
*Fighting Heart Disease
and Stroke*

Student Name _____ Date _____

Performance Guidelines	Performed
1. Establish unresponsiveness. If second rescuer is available, have him or her activate the EMS system.	
2. Open airway and try to ventilate; if still obstructed, reposition head and try to ventilate again.	
3. Give up to 5 back blows and 5 chest thrusts.	
4. Perform a tongue-jaw lift, and if you see the object, perform a finger sweep to remove it.	
5. Repeat steps 2 through 4 until effective.*	
6. If airway obstruction is not relieved after about 1 minute, activate the EMS system.	

*If victim is breathing or resumes effective breathing, place in recovery position.

Comments _____

_____

_____

Instructor _____

Circle one: Complete   Needs more practice

59

Appendix 1
Your Commonly Asked
Questions About CPR

1. **What about AIDS or hepatitis or other disease transmission during CPR?**

   Disease transmission, particularly of the AIDS and hepatitis viruses, while performing CPR is an obvious concern. The probability that a rescuer will become infected with either the AIDS or hepatitis virus as a result of performing CPR is minimal. To date, transmission of AIDS and hepatitis during mouth-to-mouth resuscitation has not been documented. If you are still concerned, face masks and shields can be used as barrier devices. These devices are placed over the victim's mouth.

   More important, remember that about 70% to 80% of respiratory and cardiac arrests occur in the home. In these situations the rescuer usually knows the victim and knows about the victim's health. A primary reason to learn CPR is for the benefit of one's family and close friends.

2. **What are the hazards of CPR?**

   Incorrect performance of CPR can cause injury to victims. Performance guidelines should be followed, and manikin practice is often useful.

   Incorrect performance of CPR may include

   - **Incorrect hand position** for chest compressions, which may cause rib fracture, xiphoid fracture, and bruising or bleeding of the liver, lung, or spleen
   - **Failure to release pressure completely between chest compressions,** which prevents the heart from filling with blood
   - **Bouncing chest compressions,** which may cause the rescuer's hands to move off the sternum
   - **Failing to compress the sternum deeply enough,** which results in inadequate blood flow to the brain and other vital organs

- **Compressing the chest too deeply,** which may cause internal injury

- **Using rescue breath volumes that are too great,** breathing too rapidly, or not having the airway opened completely, allowing gastric distention to build up, which may predispose the victim to vomiting or decrease the effectiveness of ventilation

- **Incorrect hand positions** for abdominal thrusts (the Heimlich maneuver), which may damage the internal organs

Even when CPR is performed correctly, you may hear popping noises or cracking sounds as you are compressing. If this happens, you should stop, check for proper hand position, and continue. If hand position is correct, the sounds are probably due to separation of the ribs from the sternum at the costochondral (bone-cartilage) junction, and the injury will heal after successful resuscitation. Rib fractures are possible even with correct hand position, especially in the elderly or chronically ill victim, but they will also heal. Other complications may occur despite proper CPR technique, including fracture of the sternum, lung contusions, and lacerations of the liver. These complications may be minimized by careful attention to details of performance.

Remember, not performing CPR or not applying the necessary force to the chest for fear of causing injury to the cardiac arrest victim will certainly result in the victim's death.

3. **How do I open the airway of a victim who may have a neck injury, such as the victim of an automobile accident?**

Chin lift without head tilt is the first step in opening the airway in a victim with suspected neck injury. If this is unsuccessful, the head is tilted back slowly and gently until the airway is open.

4. **What should I do if the victim vomits?**

You should turn the victim's head and body to the side so that the victim will not choke on the vomitus, then clear the airway by sweeping the mouth. A cloth (corner of clothing, handkerchief, etc) over your fingers can be used to sweep out the mouth. The victim should then be repositioned, and CPR should be continued.

5. How will I know if CPR is effective?

The compression and ventilation that you are providing for the victim should meet AHA guidelines. For example, depressing the sternum $1\frac{1}{2}$ to 2 inches should provide adequate compression for the adult. One way to assess your performance is for a second rescuer to monitor the carotid pulse while you administer CPR. A good, strong carotid or brachial pulse should be present with each compression.

Rescue breathing can be checked by watching to see if the victim's chest rises with each lung inflation. Remember, too much volume will cause stomach distention.

6. How will I know if pulse and breathing return?

The spontaneous return of pulse with or without breathing may be dramatic or subtle. If dramatic, the victim may take a big gasp of air, begin moving, or even start to regain conscious-ness. If subtle, it will be found only as you check the pulse.

This assessment is to be done after the first 4 cycles of breaths/compressions in the adult (and after 20 cycles in the child or infant) and then every few minutes.

After delivering the 2 breaths of the last cycle for the adult (or the 1 breath for the child and infant), check for pulse (reassess-ment): leave your hand on the forehead to keep the airway open, and then with two fingers of the other hand feel for the carotid pulse (in infants, the brachial pulse). If the pulse is still absent, resume CPR. If the pulse is present, check for breathing.

- If breathing is present, keep the airway open and monitor pulse and breathing. Place the victim in the recovery posi-tion to maintain an open airway.

- If breathing is absent, perform rescue breathing 12 times per minute (once every 5 seconds) for the adult and 20 times per minute (once every 3 seconds) for the child or infant, and keep checking the pulse.

7. What should I do about a "neck breather" in need of CPR?

Neck breathers are persons who have undergone surgical removal of the voice box (larynx) and have a permanent opening (stoma) that connects the airway or windpipe (trachea) directly to the skin. This is recognized by observing the opening at the base of the front of the neck.

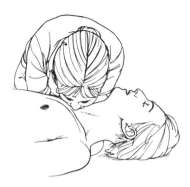

To tell whether the victim's breathing has returned, place your ear over the opening in the neck.

If rescue breathing is required, do direct mouth-to-stoma rescue breathing. For more information, contact the International Association of Laryngectomees, c/o the American Cancer Society, 1599 Clifton Rd. NE, Atlanta, GA 30329.

8. If a victim is found on a bed, how do I move him or her to the floor so that I have a hard surface under the victim's spine?

When moving a victim, protect the head and neck at all times. If you are alone and cannot move the victim, leave the victim on the bed and find something flat and firm to slide under the back to provide a hard surface.

9. What do I do for an adult who I think is having a heart attack?

The initial reaction should be to have the victim rest quietly and calmly. Both angina pectoris and heart attack are caused by too little oxygen to the heart muscle. Thus, activity should be kept to a minimum.

If chest discomfort lasts more than a few minutes, the EMS system should be activated. (Phone First!)

10. What do I do if a person takes nitroglycerin and is having chest discomfort?

Have the person rest and take the nitroglycerin as prescribed. If the chest pain persists after several doses of nitroglycerin, the EMS system should be activated.

11. **If I find a victim and I am alone, should I telephone for help first or should I immediately begin CPR?**

For the adult victim, phone first and then begin CPR. The sooner EMS arrives, the better the chance for survival of the adult because of the special skills and equipment of EMS units (Phone First!). Because children have respiratory arrests more often than cardiac arrests, begin CPR first, and if, after about 1 minute, the child has not regained spontaneous pulse and breathing, take the least time possible and phone for help (Phone Fast!).

12. **What should I do if the victim is wearing dentures?**

Leave the dentures in place if possible. This will help you make an airtight seal around the victim's mouth. Remove the dentures only if they are so loose or ill-fitting that they get in your way.

13. **What should I do to prevent stomach distention (gastric distention)?**

Distention of the stomach (air getting into the stomach) is most likely to occur when excessive pressures are used for inflation or if the airway is partially obstructed. The chance of gastric distention can be minimized by controlling the force and speed of rescue breaths: breathe slowly into the victim for $1\frac{1}{2}$ to 2 seconds each time, and check that you are not forcing breaths after the chest rises.

14. **What if the victim of complete airway obstruction is pregnant or very obese?**

The pregnant or obese victim of choking should have the same treatment as any other victim unless it is impossible to perform safe or effective abdominal thrusts because the pregnancy is advanced or the obesity is extreme. In these cases, chest thrusts should be performed rather than abdominal thrusts.

To perform chest thrusts in the conscious victim (standing or sitting):

- Stand behind the victim.
- With your arms under the victim's armpits, encircle the victim's chest.

- Place the thumb side of your fist in the middle of the breastbone. Grab your fist with the other hand.
- Perform backward thrusts until the foreign body is expelled or the victim becomes unconscious.

To perform chest thrusts in the unconscious victim (lying on a firm surface):

- Place the victim on his or her back.
- Kneel close to the victim's body.
- Use the same hand position as that for chest compressions.
- Perform each thrust decisively and distinctly, with the intent of relieving the obstruction.

15. How will I know when to start the obstructed airway sequence in a conscious choking victim?

Foreign bodies may cause either partial or complete airway obstruction. With partial airway obstruction, the victim may be capable of either "good air exchange" or "poor air exchange." With good air exchange the victim can cough forcefully, although frequently there is wheezing between coughs. As long as good air exchange continues, the victim should be allowed and encouraged to persist with spontaneous coughing and breathing efforts. At this point *do not* interfere with the victim's attempts to expel the foreign body. The victim is more likely to be able to expel the foreign body than you are at this point.

Poor air exchange may occur initially, or good air exchange may progress to poor air exchange as indicated by a weak, ineffective cough and high-pitched crowing noises while inhaling. At this point treat the partial obstruction as though it were a complete airway obstruction.

With complete airway obstruction, the victim is unable to speak, breathe, or cough. The victim also may clutch his or her neck (universal distress signal). If he or she cannot speak, *begin the obstructed airway sequence.*

16. **What should I do if I am unable to open the mouth to give rescue breaths?**

   Mouth-to-nose rescue breathing is an effective alternative to mouth-to-mouth rescue breathing.

   - Tilt the head back with one hand on the forehead.
   - With the other hand, lift the chin and close the mouth.
   - Take a deep breath, seal your lips around the nose of the victim, and blow into the nose.
   - Release the pressure on the chin to let the air out during exhalation.

17. **What are the dangers of the Heimlich maneuver?**

   There is a chance of damage to internal organs or vomiting. Your hands should be above the navel and below the xiphoid process (the tip of the sternum) for abdominal thrusts.

   In infants there is heightened concern about potential damage to internal organs from abdominal thrusts. Therefore, back blows and chest thrusts are used instead of the Heimlich maneuver.

   For chest thrusts, the hands should be above the xiphoid process.

18. **What can I do if I am a choking victim and I am alone?**

   The victim who is alone can perform the thrust on himself or herself in the following manner: press a fist into the upper abdomen with a quick upward thrust as described for the standing victim or lean forward and press the abdomen quickly over any firm object, such as a table or the back of a chair.

19. **Should I handle a drowning victim differently from any other victim?**

   Not really. After determining unresponsiveness, opening the airway, establishing breathlessness, and attempting rescue breathing, if rescue breaths do not inflate the chest, begin the obstructed airway sequence:

   - Reposition head and attempt rescue breathing.
   - If still unable to give rescue breaths, give 5 abdominal thrusts (the Heimlich maneuver).

- Use tongue-jaw lift and sweep mouth with hooked finger.
- Try to give rescue breaths.

There are cases of drowning victims, especially children, for whom successful resuscitations have taken place after 20 to 30 minutes of submersion in cold water. *Never* assume that it has been too long. Always attempt CPR. You may save a life!

20. How long can I stop CPR to move the victim?

Do not interrupt CPR for more than a few seconds for any reason except for special situations, such as transporting the victim. If it is necessary to move a victim up or down a stairway, perform effective CPR at the head or foot of the stairs, then interrupt CPR and move quickly to the next flat area, where effective CPR must be resumed.

21. For rescuers with arthritic problems of the hand and wrist or other problems that make compression difficult, how can chest compressions be done?

An acceptable alternative hand position is grasping the wrist of the hand on the chest with the hand that has been locating the lower end of the sternum.

22. How often should I retake this CPR course?

The national ECC Committee recommends retraining at least every 2 years to refresh CPR skills. Your local AHA may recommend even more frequent skill renewal. The affiliate will inform you of local suggested renewal procedures. For more information, please contact your local American Heart Association.

Appendix 2
Self-test Questions

1. **People with the early signs of a heart attack often:**
   a. panic and faint
   b. deny that they are having a heart attack
   c. drive themselves to the doctor
   d. go to sleep to relieve the pain
   Answer, p. 18

2. **It is important to know about the risk factors for heart disease because they:**
   a. indicate whether you are going to have a heart attack
   b. identify factors that may lead to heart attack
   c. scare people into quitting smoking
   d. can help you recover from a heart attack
   Answer, p. 13

3. **A person having a heart attack may say that it feels like:**
   a. "an uncomfortable pressure"
   b. "a tightness around my chest"
   c. "bad indigestion"
   d. all of the above
   Answer, p. 18

4. **The most serious danger of heart attack is:**
   a. stroke
   b. brain death
   c. severe pain in the chest
   d. cardiac arrest
   Answer, p. 2

5. **Before the rescuer attempts to resuscitate the victim by performing CPR, the following condition should exist:**
   a. brain damage
   b. dilated pupils
   c. absence of breath and pulse
   d. shallow breathing
   Answer, pp. 28, 30

6. **The most common cause of airway obstruction in the unconscious victim is:**
   a. food
   b. tongue and epiglottis
   c. mucus
   d. dentures
   Answer, p. 24

7. **The *first* thing that should be done for a collapsed victim of illness or accident is:**
   a. examine the victim's mouth for foreign bodies
   b. determine unresponsiveness
   c. perform the Heimlich maneuver
   d. open the airway
   Answer, p. 28

8. **If the airway seems obstructed after the first attempt to give rescue breaths to an unconscious victim, the rescuer should:**
   a. reposition the head and attempt rescue breaths again
   b. begin chest compressions
   c. go on to check the pulse
   d. check for foreign-body airway obstruction
   Answer, p. 37

9. **The method used for opening the airway is:**
   a. head tilt with chin lift
   b. turning the head to one side
   c. striking the victim on the back
   d. wiping out the mouth and throat
   Answer, p. 28

10. **The presence of breathing in an unconscious victim can be determined by:**
    a. checking for pupil dilation
    b. checking for discoloration of skin
    c. checking the pulse
    d. looking, listening, and feeling for air exchange
    Answer, pp. 28–29

11. **If breathing does not seem to be present after opening the airway:**
    a. begin chest compressions
    b. determine pulselessness
    c. check pupils
    d. give 2 rescue breaths
    Answer, p. 28

12. **If vomiting occurs during the resuscitative effort, the best procedure is to:**
    a. activate the EMS system
    b. stop CPR and wait for help
    c. change to mouth-to-nose rescue breathing
    d. turn victim to side, sweep out mouth, and resume resuscitation
    Answer, p. 61

13. **A rescuer's first effort to ensure that the victim's airway is open should be to:**
    a. attempt to give rescue breaths
    b. position the head properly
    c. clear foreign matter from the throat
    d. shake the victim and shout "Are you OK?"
    Answer, pp. 24, 28–29

14. **After breaths given by the rescuer, the victim will exhale by:**
    a. normal relaxation of the chest
    b. gentle pressure of the rescuer's hand on the upper chest
    c. compressions on the chest
    d. turning the victim's head to the side
    Answer, p. 29

15. **Gastric distention during CPR is caused by:**
    a. air entering the victim's stomach
    b. inadequate exhalation by the unconscious victim
    c. excessive fluids in the stomach
    d. too much chest compression force
    Answer, pp. 61, 64

16. **To determine initially whether an adult victim has a pulse, the rescuer should feel for the pulse at the:**
    a. brachial artery in the arm
    b. femoral artery in the groin
    c. carotid artery in the neck
    d. radial artery in the wrist
    Answer, p. 31

17. **Complications that may result from chest compressions even when properly performed include:**
    a. punctured lungs
    b. lacerated liver
    c. fractured ribs and sternum
    d. all of the above
    Answer, pp. 60–61

18. **To perform chest compressions on an adult, one hand is placed on top of the other with the heel of the lower hand pressing:**
   a. on the lower half of the sternum
   b. on the upper third of the sternum
   c. on the middle of the sternum
   d. on the xiphoid process
   Answer, p. 31

19. **When performing chest compressions on an adult, the sternum should be depressed:**
   a. $1/2$ to 1 inch
   b. 1 to $1\frac{1}{2}$ inches
   c. $1\frac{1}{2}$ to 2 inches
   d. 2 to $2\frac{1}{2}$ inches
   Answer, p. 31

20. **When the rescuer is alone with a pediatric arrest victim and there is no possibility that another person will arrive, the rescuer should:**
   a. activate the EMS system before opening the victim's airway
   b. do nothing and wait for help to arrive
   c. open the victim's airway, then activate the EMS system
   d. perform CPR for 1 minute, then activate the EMS system
   Answer, pp. 40, 64

21. **To determine if there is an obstructed airway in a conscious victim, the rescuer should:**
   a. ask the victim "Are you choking?"
   b. shake the victim
   c. reposition the victim
   d. perform abdominal thrusts
   Answer, pp. 34–35

22. **To perform the Heimlich maneuver for an unconscious victim, the rescuer should:**
   a. sit on the victim's ankles
   b. kneel beside the victim's chest
   c. kneel beside the victim's feet
   d. kneel astride the victim's thighs
   Answer, p. 37

23. **If a victim is coughing forcefully with a *partial* airway obstruction:**
    a. check the pulse
    b. give abdominal thrusts
    c. sweep out the mouth
    d. do not interfere
    Answer, p. 65

24. **Foreign-body obstruction of the airway in the adult usually occurs:**
    a. during sleep
    b. during eating
    c. during a heart attack
    d. during exercise
    Answer, p. 22

25. **Failure to ventilate the victim's lungs adequately can be caused by:**
    a. excessive air in the stomach
    b. inadequate head tilt
    c. lack of an airtight seal
    d. any of the above
    Answer, pp. 37, 47, 61, 64

26. **If after back blows an *infant's* airway is still obstructed:**
    a. give up to 5 abdominal thrusts
    b. give up to 5 additional back blows
    c. give up to 5 chest thrusts
    d. turn the infant upside down and shake him or her
    Answer, pp. 45–46

27. **In performing CPR, the chest of the *infant* should be compressed:**
    a. $1/2$ to 1 inch
    b. 1 to $1^1/2$ inches
    c. $1^1/2$ to 2 inches
    d. 2 to $2^1/2$ inches
    Answer, p. 44

28. **The *rate* of chest compressions in an *infant* is at least:**
    a. 60 times per minute
    b. 80 times per minute
    c. 90 times per minute
    d. 100 times per minute
    Answer, p. 44

29. **The most common cause of cardiac arrest in *infants* and *children* is:**
    a. heart attack
    b. respiratory arrest
    c. electric shock
    d. drowning
    Answer, p. 38

30. **In *infants* and *children* the *ratio* of compressions to ventilations (rescue breaths) is:**
    a. 15 compressions to 2 ventilations
    b. 15 compressions to 5 ventilations
    c. 5 compressions to 1 ventilation
    d. 5 compressions to 2 ventilations
    Answer, pp. 40, 41, 44

31. **The rescuer should check the *infant's* pulse by feeling the:**
    a. carotid pulse in the neck
    b. brachial pulse in the arm
    c. radial pulse in the wrist
    d. femoral pulse in the groin
    Answer, pp. 43, 44, 62

32. **According to guidelines of the American Heart Association, *child* CPR is performed on a victim:**
    a. under 1 year of age
    b. 1 to 8 years of age
    c. 8 to 10 years of age
    d. 10 to 12 years of age
    Answer, p. 40

33. **In performing CPR, the chest of the *child* should be compressed:**
    a. $1/2$ to 1 inch
    b. 1 to $1^1/_2$ inches
    c. $1^1/_2$ to 2 inches
    d. 2 to $2^1/_2$ inches
    Answer, pp. 40, 41

34. **Rescue breathing for a *child* with a pulse should be performed:**
    a. 10 times per minute
    b. 12 times per minute
    c. 15 times per minute
    d. 20 times per minute
    Answer, p. 41

Appendix 3
Legal and Ethical Issues

Recognition is given for successful completion of a CPR course based on criteria established by the American Heart Association. It does not imply licensure or warrant future performance.

• • •

There is no instance known in which a layperson who has performed CPR has been sued successfully. Good Samaritan laws in most states specifically protect professionals and laypersons performing CPR "in good faith." Under most Good Samaritan laws, laypersons are protected if they perform CPR even if they have had no formal training.

All citizens should learn to perform CPR well enough to sustain the life of the victim until professional emergency medical treatment becomes available unless such performance would pose a medical or emotional danger to themselves.

• • •

As a rescuer acting in good faith, you should remember that once CPR is begun, you should stop only when one of the following occurs:

- The victim recovers (regains pulse and breathing)
- Another trained person takes over
- You are too exhausted to continue
- A valid DNR (Do-Not-Resuscitate) order is presented to the rescuer

The Patient Self-determination Act of 1991 was intended to support the rights of patients to make decisions about their medical care and to make advance directives. Physicians and families should talk with patients about their preferences regarding CPR in various clinical settings. For more information, contact your physician or hospital.

Appendix 4
Glossary of Heart Terms

Angina Pectoris — A condition in which the heart muscle receives an insufficient blood supply, causing temporary pain in the chest and often in the left arm and shoulder, usually during exercise or when the patient is emotionally upset.

Artery — Blood vessel that carries blood away from the heart to the various parts of the body.

Atherosclerosis — A condition in which the inner layers of artery walls are made thick and irregular by deposits of a fatty substance. The internal channel of arteries becomes narrowed, and blood supply is reduced.

Blood Pressure — The force of pressure exerted by the heart in pumping blood; the pressure of blood in the arteries.

Capillaries — The smallest blood vessels, which distribute oxygenated blood to the cells of the body.

Cardiac — Pertaining to the heart.

Cardiac Arrest — The heart stops beating.

Cardiopulmonary Resuscitation (CPR) — A combination of chest compressions and mouth-to-mouth rescue breathing used during cardiac and respiratory arrest to keep oxygenated blood flowing to the brain until advanced life support can be initiated.

Cardiovascular — Pertaining to the heart and blood vessels.

Cholesterol (dietary) — A fatlike substance found in animal tissue.

Circulatory System — The heart and blood vessels (arteries, veins, and capillaries).

Coronary Arteries — Arteries arising from the aorta, circling the surface of the heart, and conducting blood to the heart muscle.

Coronary Care Unit (CCU) — An in-hospital specialized facility or emergency mobile unit equipped with monitoring devices, staffed with trained personnel, and designed to treat coronary patients.

Coronary Occlusion — An obstruction or narrowing of one of the coronary arteries that hinders blood flow to part of the heart muscle. See "Heart Attack."

Coronary Thrombosis — Formation of a clot in one of the arteries that conduct blood to the heart muscle. Also called "coronary occlusion."

Diabetes Mellitus — A chronic disease of carbohydrate metabolism, usually due to an abnormal production or release of insulin in the body.

Heart Attack — A nonspecific term usually referring to complete blockage of a diseased coronary artery by a blood clot, resulting in the death of the heart muscle cells supplied by that artery. "Myocardial infarction" is a more specific term for what is usually meant by "heart attack."

High Blood Pressure (Hypertension) — Persistent elevation of blood pressure above the normal range.

Hypertension — See "High Blood Pressure."

Myocardial Infarction — See "Heart Attack."

Myocardium — Heart muscle.

Nitroglycerin — Drug that causes dilation of blood vessels, often used in the treatment of angina pectoris.

Occluded Artery — One in which blood flow has been impaired by a blockage.

Pulmonary — Pertaining to the lungs.

Stroke — A sudden and often severe attack caused by an insufficient supply of blood to part of the brain. Older terms for stroke are "apoplexy," "cerebrovascular accident," and "cerebral vascular accident."

Vascular — Pertaining to the blood vessels.

Vein — Any one of a series of vessels of the vascular system that carries blood from various parts of the body back to the heart.

Appendix 5
Public Access Defibrillation
and Automated External Defibrillators

Automated External Defibrillators Can Make Early Defibrillation Easy

Early defibrillation saves lives. The main problem for early defibrillation is getting a defibrillator to the victim in just a few minutes, and you must have a person trained to operate it. Automated external defibrillators (AEDs) are a major advance in resuscitation. You have to have lots of training to use other defibrillators (called manual defibrillators), but you can use AEDs after only a little training. This means that many more people can use an AED, and they can help make early defibrillation a reality.

In AEDs the work is done by a computer. When an AED is attached to a victim, it rapidly analyzes the electrical activity of the victim's heart and then decides if a shock is needed. AEDs are easy to use, they are very accurate, and they have saved many lives. However, a challenge still remains: to get AEDs to victims of cardiac arrest.

Public Access Defibrillation

Public access defibrillation is a recent idea developed by the American Heart Association. Public access defibrillation allows AEDs to be used by a much larger number of rescuers than in the past. For example, in many communities firefighters and police officers can now use AEDs. By using AEDs quickly and safely, they have improved survival rates for out-of-hospital cardiac arrest.

Early defibrillation would reach even more people if lay rescuers could use AEDs in the home and workplace. In places where large numbers of people gather, such as office buildings, hotels, malls, stadiums, and public buildings, AEDs should be available for lay rescuers to use before EMS personnel arrive. This strategy could help in cities where traffic congestion often delays the response of EMS personnel. It could also help in rural areas where EMS personnel take longer to arrive.

The airline industry has begun to carry AEDs on regular flights. During the next few years more industries concerned about safety will probably follow the example of the airlines by starting early defibrillation programs.

Saving More Lives in the Community

To save more lives, early defibrillation must become the standard of care for all. Some communities have made progress toward this goal, but many still need major improvement.

Defibrillation once was a skill reserved for highly trained emergency care providers, but AEDs and public access defibrillation challenge that notion. It is now possible for minimally trained lay rescuers to operate an AED, and the price of AEDs has become reasonable. The challenge for the coming decade is to determine how widely AEDs can be placed.

Additional research is required to determine how far public access defibrillation can go toward saving lives.